Healthy

Handbook
Over 50s Edition

Your Guide to Getting the Vitamins You Need as You Age

RON KNESS

Contents

Disclaimer

This publication is for informational purposes only and is not intended as medical advice. Medical advice should always be obtained from a qualified medical professional for any health conditions or symptoms associated with them.

Every possible effort has been made in preparing and researching this material. We make no warranties with respect to the accuracy, applicability of its contents or any omissions.

See your healthcare professional before starting any diet, health or exercise program!

Introduction

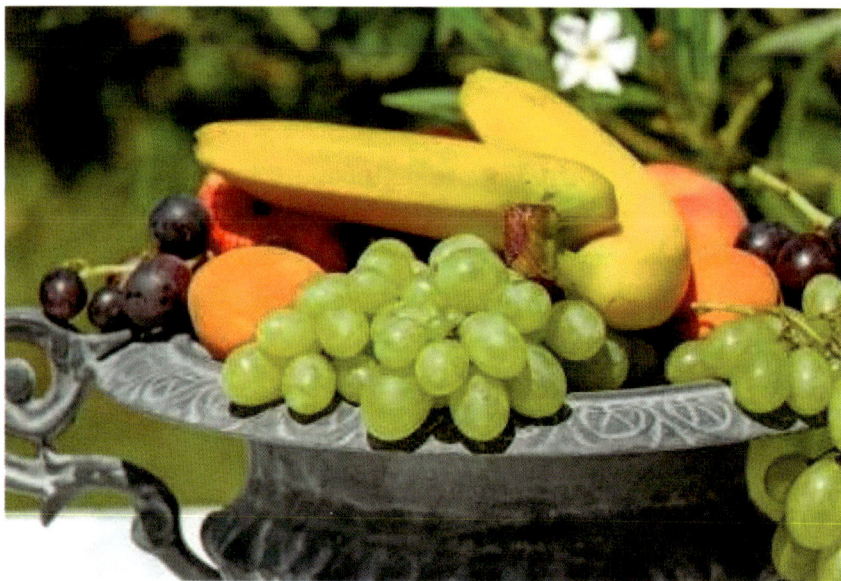

Vitamins are incredibly important nutrients. After all, many of us take vitamins every morning, emphasize eating foods full of vitamins, and will choose something that is advertised as having vitamins before we choose a different product. So, vitamins are very, very good. We all know this, but rarely do we understand why. Vitamins are organic substances that we need teeny tiny amounts of to make sure our bodies are running properly.

And we need to eat them to get enough of them. Unlike fat, or glucose, which we can synthesize replacements for, our ability to make our own vitamins is little to none. In most cases we simply can't make the vitamins we need, and absolutely need to eat them. And even in rare cases where our bodies make or recycle their own vitamins, we usually make just enough to keep us going through harsh times.

Take, for example, Arctic explorers and Arctic inhabitants. The explorers suffered Vitamin C deficiency, but only months after stopping having Vitamin C. The inhabitants rarely if ever suffered it due to their intake of a few key foods, because their bodies recycled Vitamin C as much as possible. But if we stop eating any vitamin for long enough, we will start to become deficient and ill.

So how can we make sure we are getting enough variety of vitamins, so that we are healthy and happy? The most basic way to do this is to eat a wide range of fruits and vegetables, but over time you may find that your vitamin levels go down, even though your diet stays the same.

Getting Enough Vitamins Gets Harder as You Age

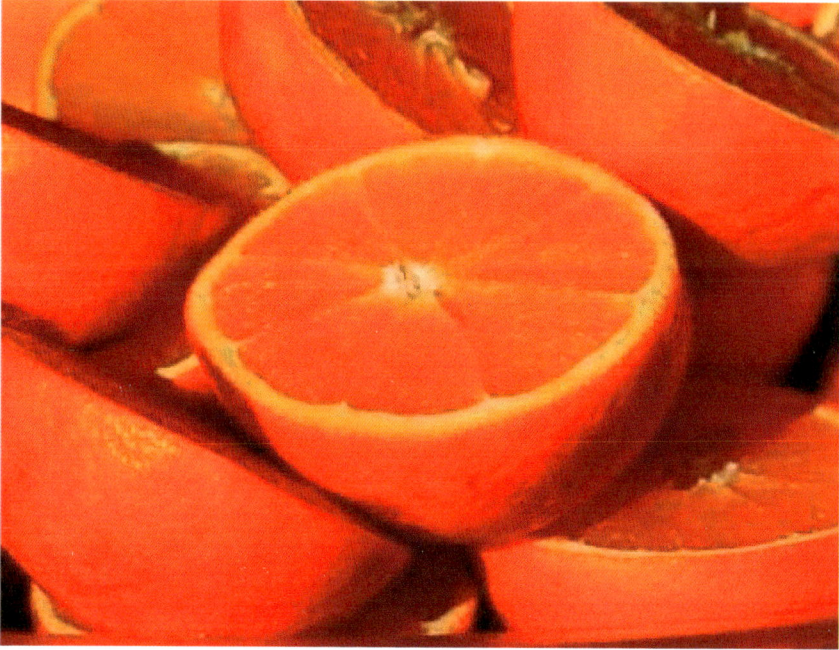

When we are younger, our diet is often more than enough for providing the nutrients we need. The first and biggest reason for this is quite simply the number of calories we can eat. When we are younger, we eat far more calories because we need far more calories. In part, this is due to the fact that younger people often do more.

It may not seem like a lot, but even the daily walk to and from the car or train station, and milling around the office, will burn some calories. And if you were very physically active in your youth? Then you may expect a more dramatic reduction in the number of calories you need.

But there are physical changes too. For example, for women entering the menopause the loss of their cycles means two things. First of all, they do not need as many calories, as they are not growing and shedding a womb lining every month. But secondly, as there is no risk of pregnancy they no longer need to carry as much body fat. This means that menopausal and postmenopausal women will need to lose weight and be slimmer to be healthier. *And* they will not need a calorie boost once a month either. Which naturally means eating fewer calories.

As we grow older we also find that our muscle tissue degrades. This is because after a short spike, a hormone called myostatin, that is responsible for maintaining our hormones, declines sharply. So, our bodies need to work harder and harder to hold onto the muscle they already have. Testosterone, another important hormone for muscle development and retention, also drops slowly as we grow older. And due to mobility issues and pains, many older people cannot keep up the level of exercise they once did, resulting in muscle wasting away.

The end result of losing muscle tissue is an even greater reduction in the number of calories we can afford to eat without gaining weight. Fat and bone and other tissues are very metabolically lazy. They don't do a lot, so they don't burn many calories. Muscle, on the other hand, burns more calories than fat even when we're not using it.

So, losing a mere 5 pounds of muscle could mean losing 36 calories a day. Which doesn't sound like a lot, but over 97 days that adds up to an extra pound of fat. Or an extra four pounds of fat in a year. So, this is something we need to watch closely, especially when added to the other things already reducing out metabolism.

The final effect of all these reductions in our calorific needs is remarkable. If we are a perfectly average, moderately active person until the age of fifty, we will need 2000 calories up until that point. But then, from some point in our fifties onward, we lose a whole 200 calories, meaning we need to suddenly eat 1800 to maintain our weight. The effect is more dramatic for women, and for people leading sedentary lives.

An average height and build woman who is moderately active only needs 1750 to maintain a healthy weight in the first place, and after 50 she will need 1550. And an average height and build man who is sedentary only needs 1800 until the age of 50, and 1600 after that. And an average height and build woman who is sedentary? She could be burning as little as 1500 calories in the first place, and need a meagre 1300 after the age of 50. Let alone people who are below average height or predisposed to being skinny.

And those spare 200 calories, if we don't cut them out, have a terrible impact on our wellbeing, adding an extra 21 pounds, or one and a half stone, every single year. The end result is that the diet that was great for us in our 20s and 30s, and not a problem in our 40s, can suddenly become a weight-gain recipe in our 50s. And many of us will react to this weight gain by dramatically reducing the amount we eat.

The reason this is a threat to our vitamin intake is simple: The number of micronutrients you get from food depends on how much food you are eating. Oranges may have 100% of our recommended vitamin C in 115 grams, or four ounces, but 1.5kg of fries, or three pounds, also has 100% of our recommended vitamin C. Naturally we probably never ate three pounds of fries a day, even in our youth.

But for example, Michael Phelps, the Olympic swimmer, on his 12,000 calorie athlete's diet, could make fries 1/3 of his diet and get enough vitamin C. The point is: even rubbish foods have *some* vitamins in them. And when we are younger we are more able to eat huge piles of rubbish foods, so we scrape just enough vitamins from ice-cream, burgers, and cakes to keep us healthy. But as we grow older, we simply cannot keep eating so much food. And as we reduce the amount of food we eat, we can suddenly go from "getting by" to "serious lack of vitamins".

Of course, not all of this is automatic. You don't *have* to suffer such a severe drop in your calorific needs as you grow older. But you need to work very hard to keep burning the same number of calories you once used to burn effortlessly. Exercising regularly obviously burns calories, so taking up a few more activities as you enter your 50s is a great way of consuming the same number of calories and keeping your nutrient intake up.

Furthermore, by staying more active you encourage your body to hold onto its muscle mass, which burns more calories. Thanks to these efforts, you could continue eating the same number of calories, the same foods, and the same number of vitamins in your 50s as in your 30s.

As We Get Older, We Need More Vitamins

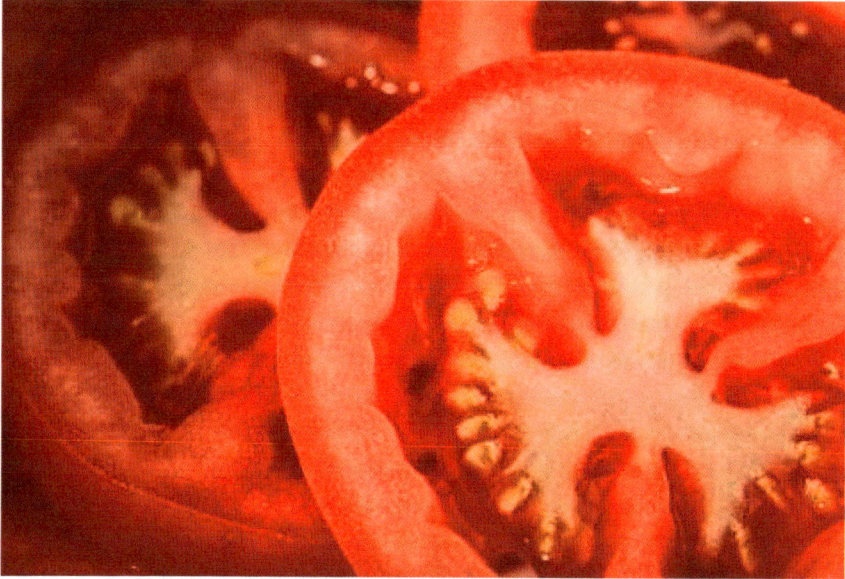

Yes, unfortunately it's not quite as simple as "work out more and keep eating the way you used to." When we are younger we aren't only able to eat a lot more food, making up our micronutrient intakes by the sheer volume of food we can eat. When we are younger we also absorb, synthesize and recycle vitamins very well. This means that as we grow older we will need to eat more and more vitamins, and higher and higher quality vitamins, to get the exact same results as in our youth.

When we are younger, nutrient absorption is at its highest and most efficient. This is because all the cells in our body are working much harder to rip nutrients out of food. We get upset guts far less commonly in our youth, for example.

Many people can go their whole youth not knowing they are lactose intolerant, or allergic to gluten, just because their guts are so strong and healthy. Meanwhile, as we grow older not only do we find pre-existing stomach and gut problems are coming to the surface, but we experience new ones as well.

As we grow older it is common to find we lose the ability to digest alliums like onions and garlic, develop reflux during meals, can't digest as much fat, need to take fiber supplements or high-fiber foods to stay regular, and cannot eat so much fruit or sweets any more. This is because our gut transit is unpredictable, our enzymes are reduced, and our gut bacteria is out of balance. So whereas a younger person may be able to get all their Vitamin A from a few carrots, an older person may need to eat a more digestible source, like liver pate, to get enough.

When we are younger vitamin synthesis is at its most powerful. Unlike many other animals, humans actually cannot truly synthesize more than one vitamin. Vitamin D can be completely produced by our bodies in response to sunlight. This is the only true synthesis of vitamins we perform. However, we *can* produce additional vitamins from foods we are eating. How?

Simple: our gut bacteria. The bacteria that live in our guts are naturally single cells that are made up of nutrients. When they digest certain foods, like fiber or resistant starch, they will release some nutrients. And when they die, they will release all the nutrients in their own cell walls. This means that if humans eat the right foods, we can get vitamins not from our own synthesis, but from the syntheses performed by our gut bacteria.

And, as we have mentioned, younger people have healthier, more effective guts than older people. This means that whereas a younger person may be able to rely on their gut bacteria for B vitamins, for example, an older person may get little to no vitamins at all from their guts.

When we are younger we are far, far more capable of recycling vitamins from waste. Ordinarily, our bodies will release excess vitamins in our urine, store them in our fat, or break them down for different uses in different processes. But if we just aren't eating a certain vitamin and our body levels get critical, our bodies have an ace up their sleeves. They can take some of this wasted vitamin material and reuse it for other important vitamin tasks.

We can't do this indefinitely, as most vitamins are in some way broken down or consumed as we use them, but this process greatly lengthens the amount of time it takes for us to become deficient. However, as our metabolisms become less efficient as we grow older, we are more prone to wasting these surplus vitamins. The same way a drop in myostatin means our bodies do not hold onto muscle as well after the age of 50, a drop in various other hormones means our bodies do not hold onto vitamins well after a certain age either.

And finally, when we are younger we don't really need so many nutrients. During early childhood, we need a lot proportionately to our body size, because of how much we are growing, but as a total it's a teeny tiny dose, smaller than the average adult needs. And during adulthood we don't need much because our bodies are very effective at maintaining themselves. However, as we grow older a part of our cells called telomeres grow shorter and shorter.

These are the little arms at the end of our chromosomes which protect them from degrading, and they are very important.

When they are long and strong and healthy, they stop our chromosomes from malfunctioning. But the effects of oxidation caused by free radicals as we grow older will slowly wear down our telomeres, making them shorter and shorter. This means our chromosomes are more likely to malfunction.

And what do our chromosomes do? They tell our cells how to grow. Our chromosomes tell us what sex we will be, how we are meant to look, how many white blood cells our bone marrow needs to make, etc. So, when they are damaged and malfunctioning, it's a bit like having a computer bug. All of a sudden, cells start dividing the wrong way, or doing the wrong jobs. They mutate, which leads to things like the development of cancer and autoimmune conditions, loss of pigment in our hair, and loss of function in some organs.

Many of the vitamins we need act as antioxidants. This means they reverse the damage done by free radicals and preserve the length of our telomeres. This means our chromosomes are protected against mutation and we are far less likely to suffer cancer, autoimmune conditions, and other ailments. This is less relevant when we are younger as our telomeres are long and our chromosomes are strong. But we can't fight off all free radicals for ever and ever.

As we grow older our telomeres slowly shorten, no matter how hard we try and preserve them. This means that when we are younger we need fewer vitamins to keep our bodies in order, but as we grow older we need more and more.

The benefits of increasing our vitamin intake as we grow older are meaningful because they affect every cell in our bodies. Every cell in our bodies multiplies, and every cell in our bodies has telomeres. Eating more vitamins as we grow older therefore protects every single cell in our bodies against the effects of ageing, halting and even reversing brain damage, osteoporosis, renal failure, liver disease, etc.

Different Vitamins Are Absorbed and Handled In Different Ways

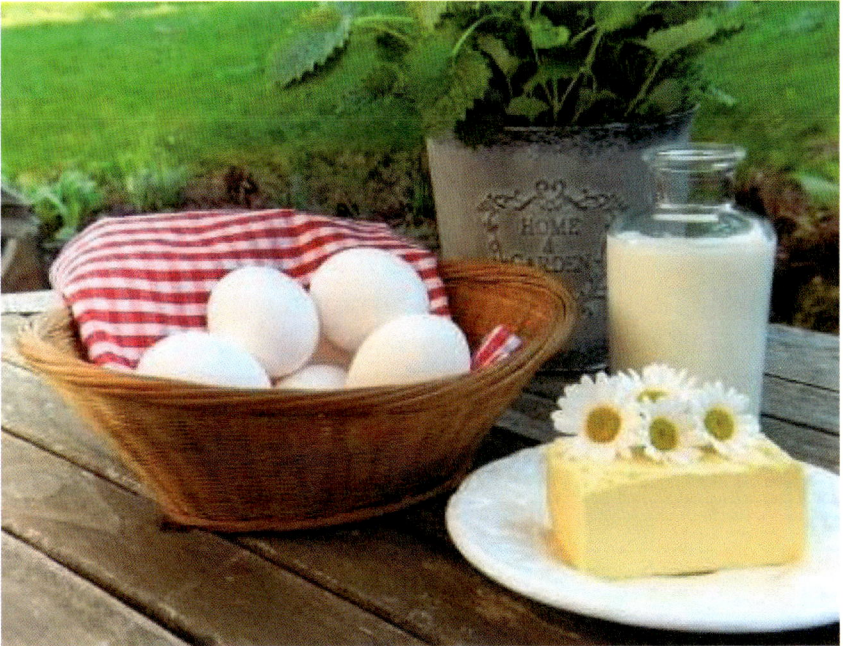

It is vital to understand that vitamins can't actually be absorbed on their own. They need to be dissolved in something to make them digestible. Some vitamins are best absorbed in fat, others in water. This means that you need to consume some vitamins with food or even a few drops of oil, whereas others are better dissolved in water. In their natural forms, the foods we eat have the right vitamins in the right places.

For example, fruits are rich in vitamin C and also rich in water, which helps carry it. Whereas liver is rich in vitamin A and also rich in fat, which transports it.

However, some foods and many supplements may have a vitamin without anything to carry it. For example, carrots are rich in a vitamin A precursor, but have no fat, dried fruit has vitamin C and no water, and you can eat powdered vitamin E, which is useless without fat. The simplest way of ensuring you get enough nutrients is to not eat too many dry foods, to drink a glass of water before or after every meal, and to ensure you eat enough healthy, varied fats.

The ones best absorbed in fat can also be stored very conveniently by the body. These vitamins can be dissolved into our own body fats and preserved for months or even years. This also comes with the inconvenient side effect that it is very easy to reach a toxic level of these vitamins. All vitamins have a toxic level, but for fat soluble ones, it is very realistic that we may reach that level by accident, even just eating a normal diet. This is especially true for meat eaters, as the fats from animal products are the easiest to digest, meaning that all trapped vitamins could easily be absorbed.

The ones best absorbed in water are much harder for our bodies to store and build a reserve of. This means we are at little to no risk of overdosing on water soluble vitamins, but also that we are at very high risk of running out of these vitamins. However, by design, they are also the ones we recycle best and need the least of. The key here is consistency. You can't go from eating vitamin C every day to eating none and expect your body to recycle it well. But if you get into a habit, your body can predict your needs much more easily and make sure to recycle enough vitamin C.

Certain vitamins and minerals also interact to improve each other's absorption. For instance, vitamin C and iron are best absorbed in each other's company, whereas vitamin D, vitamin E, and calcium all work together to ensure and develop bone health. It is important to learn which vitamins and minerals belong together, whether you are planning meals or taking supplements. When you know what nutrients, you need to eat together and where they are you can avoid accidental low vitamin levels.

Every vitamin has a vital function

To get the most out of our vitamins, we need to truly understand them. You can't know whether you are deficient in a vitamin, or have had way too much of it, if you don't know what it does, how much you need, and where you can find it. These handy notes ought to guide you in the right direction and help you make informed decisions about your diet and supplement regime. For each vitamin, we also cover when you should consider supplements, what you need to be careful about and if the vitamin is fat or water soluble.

At the end of the book, we will know a lot more about vitamins and minerals and as a result can control our health better as we age. Let's get started!

Vitamin A

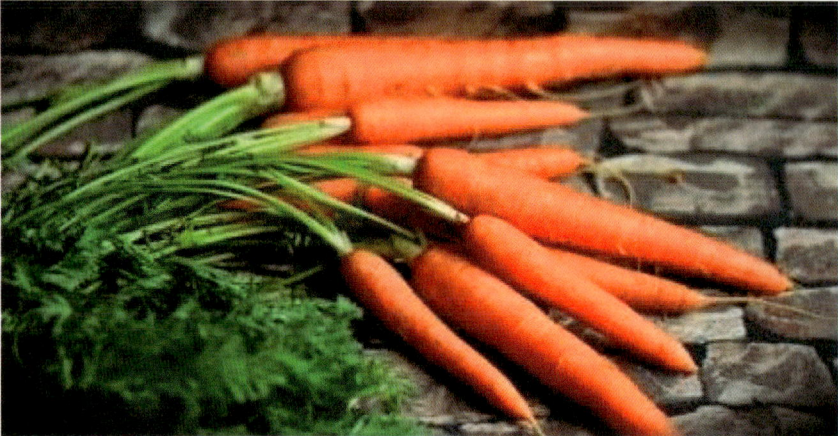

Soluble type: fat.

What does it do?

Vitamin A is key for protecting our eyesight by building networks between the eye and brain, boosts our immune system in a healthy way which includes fighting cancer and autoimmune conditions, reduces inflammation, and improves the youthfulness and health of our cells, making us look and feel younger.

How does it help people over the age of 50?

Vitamin A is a powerful antioxidant, and for that reason it helps improve all over health and slows down, sometimes even reverses, the effects of ageing.

However, vitamin A's specific benefits are also very important for people over the age of 50, when eyesight and the immune system begin to suffer.

What amount should I aim for?

Women should aim for 750mcg a day, and men for 900mcg a day. However, as this vitamin stores well, you can average this out. If you have a lot one day, have less the next, or if you haven't had much for a week, have a couple of slightly higher days.

When do I know I'm having enough?

Vitamin A deficiency, when it becomes dangerous, is very obvious to even someone who is not a medical professional. Loss of eyesight, loss of bone density, repeat UTIs, etc., are common side effects of a severe vitamin A deficiency.

Mild deficiency is less obvious. In situations where you are receiving the bare minimum, but not enough for the full health benefits, you will notice worse vision than usual, and a certain lifelessness and loss of color in your skin and hair.

On the other hand, a vitamin A overdose is a very serious, sometimes even life-threatening condition. It causes irritability, confusion, loss of appetite, vomiting, and hair loss. If you start feeling these symptoms, see your doctor immediately.

What foods can I find it in?

There are two main types of vitamin A: retinol and beta carotene. Retinol is vitamin A from animal sources, and is identical to the vitamin A in our bodies, so we don't need to process or convert it. Beta carotene is a vitamin A precursor, that is to say, it's something which turns into vitamin A inside our bodies. Some of the top food sources of retinol include beef liver, fish and dairy. Some of the best food sources of beta carotene are carrots, green leafy vegetables and sweet potatoes.

When should I consider supplements?

Because vitamin A is a fat-soluble vitamin, if you have any trouble absorbing fats you may need to consider a supplement. This is because vitamin A needs to be dissolved in fats so as to be carried around our bodies. In rare cases where fat absorption is impossible due to a weak gut or pancreas, a routine injection may be considered.

What do I need to be careful about?

Vitamin A overdoses are very easy to trigger and have very serious health consequences. In a "wild" situation, humans would never risk vitamin A overdose. In fact, in most poor societies it is unheard of, with deficiency being the biggest risk. This is because there are only two ways to overdose on vitamin A. The first is by supplementation. Eating large amounts of retinol supplements will cause you to overdose. And the second is by living largely off organ meats.

In a natural environment, we would eat much more muscle than organ meat, and much, much more beta carotene than retinol. Beta carotene is almost impossible to overdose on, as it needs to be converted to vitamin A and our bodies will stop when they have enough. But in the modern world we can easily eat plate after plate of pâté and end up with a vitamin A overdose. So, if you show any signs at all, discontinue vitamin supplementation, avoid eating offal, and consult with your doctor.

Vitamin B1, Thiamine

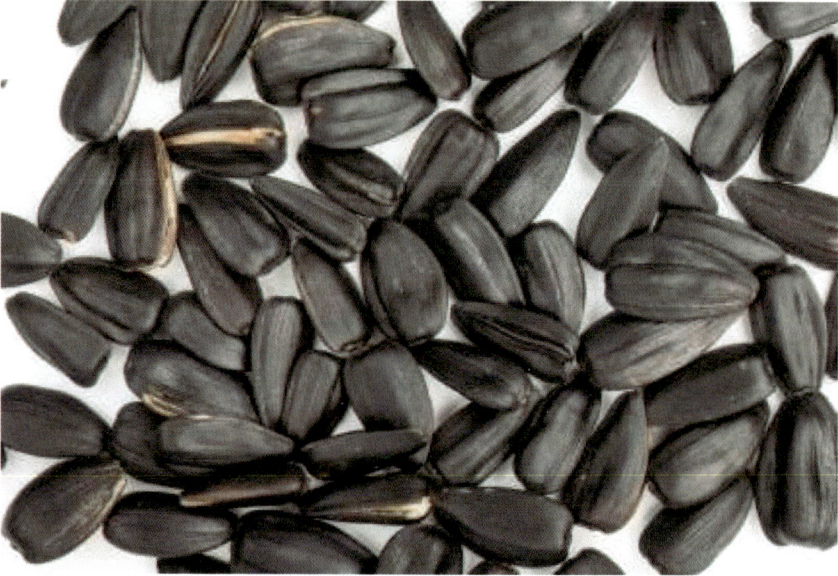

Soluble type: water.

What does it do?

Thiamine is crucial for energy and works by changing glucose and ketones into ATP, a very well broken-down product that our cells can actually burn. Almost every cell in your entire body uses vitamin B1.

How does it help people over the age of 50?

As we grow older our energy levels decline, so maintaining this energy is essential. If you find yourself feeling generally lethargic and that your mood is low, but you aren't suffering from any other physical ailments, it's possible that your ATP levels have dropped. Adding more vitamin B1 could help improve your ATP creation and give you an energy boost.

What amount should I aim for?

An intake of 1.2mg per day for men and 1.1mg per day for women is recommended, although you can go as high as three times this amount without trouble. You need to consume at least the basic 1.1-1.2mg every day, as being water soluble it is not stored well.

When do I know I'm having enough?

A serious vitamin B1 deficiency is not massively obvious, particularly if you have other conditions. This is because the key symptoms are weakness, fatigue, and signs of nerve damage like shaking hands, weight loss, and loss of memory. A deeper investigation may find that the sufferer has psychotic episodes, a swollen heart, or serious digestive problems.

Early or mild vitamin B1 deficiency is marked by a sudden loss of memory, a drop in mood, lower energy, and sudden weight loss. At this stage, it is very important to see a doctor as the later symptoms can be subtle, or hidden by early ones.

There have been very few confirmed cases of a vitamin B1 overdose. This is because it is water soluble and therefore any excess amounts of vitamin B1 is flushed out in our urine, preventing any damage. Not much is absorbed from supplements, either, so it is most likely absorbed on demand, rather than all in one go.

What foods can I find it in?

Most diets, especially in developed nations, are very rich in vitamin B1. The richest sources are plant proteins, yeasts, and organ meats. The very best source is nutritional yeast, but beans nuts, and seeds all provide almost 100% of your RDA in half a cup. However, you can also access a lot from eating two servings of liver per day.

When should I consider supplements?

You only need supplements if you are deficient in vitamin B1, which is very rare in developed nations. However, it still happens, usually because of undernourishment or drinking too much alcohol, sometimes both together. For this reason, it is essential to eat enough foods, to eat enough foods high in vitamin B1, and to not drink often, or too much.

What do I need to be careful about?

Although vitamin B1 deficiency is very rare, if you follow a special diet and have eliminated legumes, grains, nuts, seeds, and/or animal products from your diet, you are at risk of deficiency. If your diet is low carb, or largely involves fresh fruit and vegetables, you may not be eating enough vitamin B1.

Vitamin B2, Riboflavin

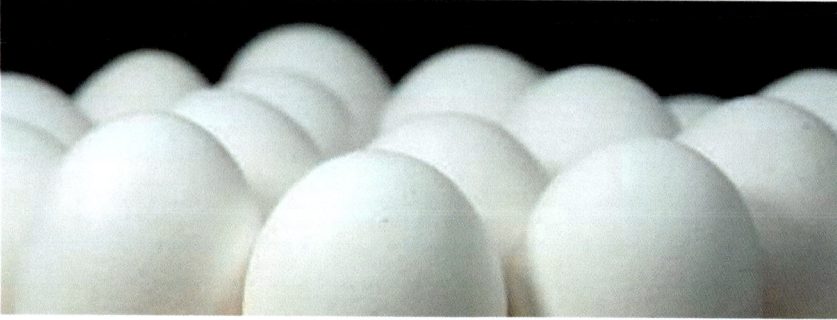

Soluble type: water.

What does it do?

Vitamin B2 plays its part in energy levels as well, improving our metabolism and ensuring our blood cells stay healthy. Vitamin B2 also plays a role in transforming glucose and ketones into ATP, to fuel our cells. This means that vitamin B2 helps ensure we have enough red blood cells and fuel to recover from illness and injury.

How does it help people over the age of 50?

As people over the age of 50 often have compromised immune systems and weaker bones and muscles, illness and injury are commonplace. By keeping your vitamin B2 levels high you won't prevent illness or injury, but you will recover faster.

What amount should I aim for?

The recommended amount is 1.3mg per day for men and 1.1mg per day for women. However, many older people suffer complaints that mean they need to eat a higher dose of it. Because it is water soluble it is not readily stored, so you will need to eat some every day, and even thought it isn't necessary to eat the exact amount every day, you must average your 1.1-1.3mg per day over the course of a week to make sure it doesn't drop too low.

When do I know I'm having enough?

Vitamin B2 deficiency is very rare in developed nations, but due to poor diet or other health concerns, it can happen. A severe deficiency in vitamin B2 leads to anemia, above all. The most serious symptoms and signs of anemia include mouth sores and cracked lips, inflammation under the skin especially on the face, a sore tongue and a lost ability to taste certain things, and a swollen nose, throat, and mouth, like when you have a cold.

When you have a minor vitamin B2 deficiency you will experience these symptoms, but only slightly. So, you may notice water retention, that you have more mouth ulcers than usual, or that food does not taste as good. A minor case of depression may occur as well.

Vitamin B2 overdose is unheard of, as if you eat too much your body will dispose of any surplus through your urine. This is because it is a water-soluble vitamin.

What foods can I find it in?

The very best sources of vitamin B2 are animal products. Meat and organ meats, high protein dairy like cheeses and Greek yogurt, and eggs are all excellent sources. For people on a vegan diet, green leafy vegetables and legumes are your best sources, and some nuts, like almonds, can add quite a bit too, though you'd have to eat them by the cupful. Seaweed is one of the very best plant-based sources of this vitamin.

When should I consider supplements?

If you suffer frequent headaches, vitamin B2 supplements have been shown to decrease symptoms and pain and shorted the duration of the headache. This is even true for migraines. And if you eat a plant-based diet and show symptoms of severe deficiency, a daily supplement could help.

What do I need to be careful about?

If you have anemia, migraines, eye conditions, hyperthyroidism, or hypothyroidism, a normal amount of vitamin B2 may not be enough to keep you healthy. This is because your condition means you don't use all the vitamin B2 which you absorb, so you need a higher dose to get the job done.

Vitamin B3, Niacin

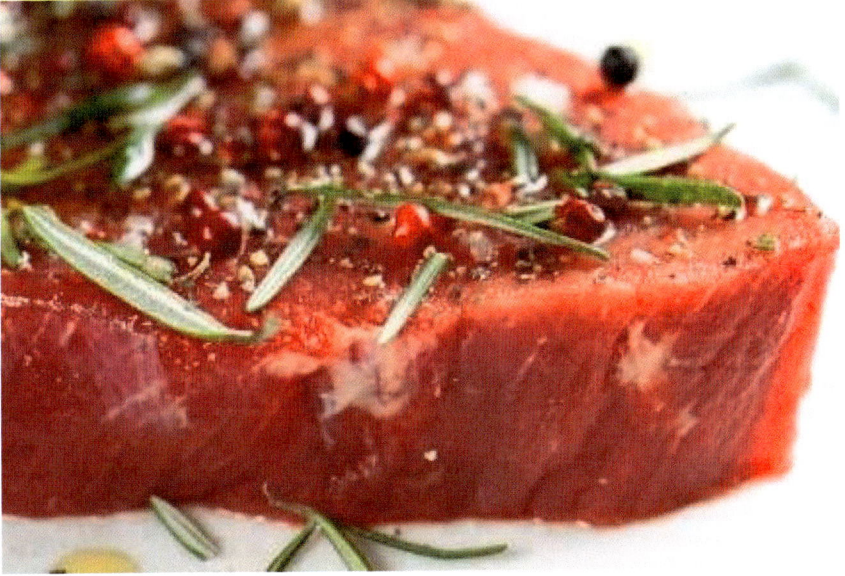

Soluble type: water.

What does it do?

Vitamin B3 has been found to successfully treat a wide range of ailments. Whether these ailments are natural and vitamin B3 is helping alleviate them, or these ailments are actually signs of a vitamin B3 deficiency which wild humans would not experience, is not known. However, it has been found to improve health all round, especially where our cardiovascular system is concerned.

How does it help people over the age of 50?

As we pass the age of fifty, our cardiovascular system becomes slowly degraded. This is why at this age the most common causes of death concern the heart. Eating enough vitamin B3 can help keep our cardiovascular system in peak condition, fighting high cholesterol, atherosclerosis, elevated blood pressure, and heart failure, expanding our lives.

What amount should I aim for?

Women should aim for 14 milligrams a day, and men for 16. However, if you suffer high blood cholesterol or high blood pressure you may benefit from consuming 2 or 3 grams a day.

When do I know I'm having enough?

Vitamin B3 deficiency is very uncommon in developed countries. However severe cases involve the development of skin rashes, severe digestive complications up to and including bloody diarrhea, and dementia symptoms. Some people will suffer sudden cognitive decline combined with manic depressive symptoms and psychoses. Fortunately, a supplement can reverse all this damage in most cases.

Minor vitamin B3 deficiency starts with swelling in the mouth and nose, as well as the genital areas. You may experience a sudden onset of mouth ulcers and find your skin is dry and develops rashes or sores. Heartburn, stomach cramps, constipation or diarrhea, and nausea are all very common as your deficiency progresses.

Vitamin B3 overdoses are possible, unlike vitamin B1 and B2 overdoses. It has been found that when someone consumes too much B3 they suffer headaches and dizziness, coinciding with episodes of low blood pressure. In short: the very thing that makes it good for us can also be bad for us, if we are predisposed to low blood pressure or if we supplement too much. Vitamin B3 overdose from natural sources has not been reported.

What foods can I find it in?

Organ meats are your single best source of vitamin B3, with a single portion of liver providing 90% of what you will need. Most muscle meats are also very rich in vitamin B3, making it easy for most omnivores to meet their basic requirements without even trying. On a plant based diet, large volumes of sunflower seeds and split peas could make up the shortfall, though you would be looking at two cups of sunflower seeds a day for your bare minimum.

When should I consider supplements?

If you are on a plant based diet and not able to eat that many vitamin B3 rich foods, or if you have high blood pressure or cholesterol and your doctor advises it, consider a supplement.

What do I need to be careful about?

If you suffer diabetes, gallbladder disease, liver disease, or gout, then you should not supplement niacin, and may find foods high in niacin worsen your symptoms. For people with these conditions, it is not wise to increase niacin intake unless guided by a doctor. Although natural niacin will not cause an overdose, it can still interfere with our blood sugar in such a way that our symptoms can snowball, causing irreversible damage.

Vitamin B5, Pantothenic Acid

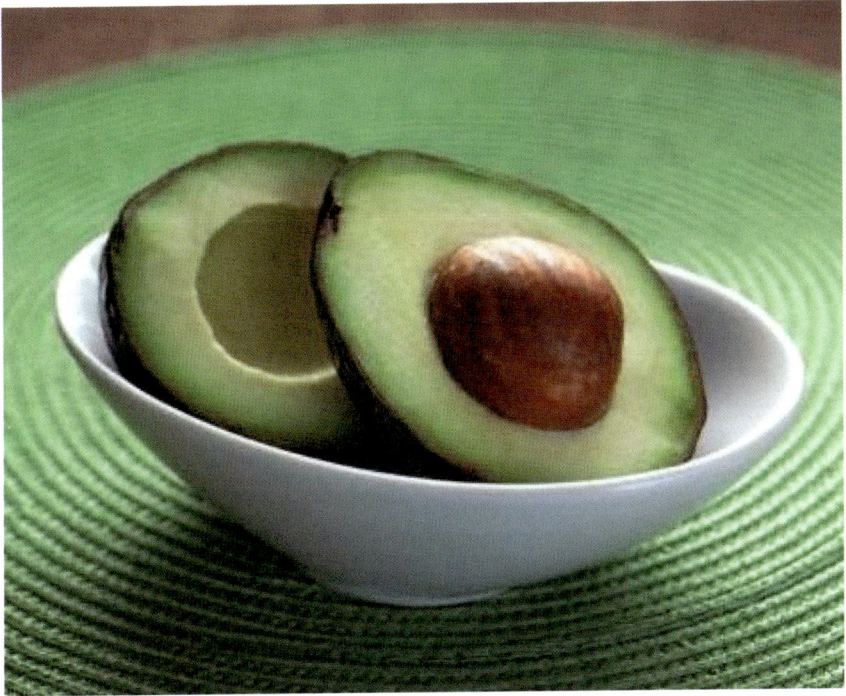

Soluble type: water.

What does it do?

As well as the usual benefits that B vitamins provide, such as balancing blood sugar, converting glucose and ketones to ATP, and improving immune function, vitamin B5 plays a unique role in reducing bad cholesterol and alleviating pain, mostly through its hormone-balancing properties.

How does it help people over the age of 50?

As we grow older, high cholesterol, physical pain, and hormonal imbalances are common complaints. For women exiting the menopause, hormonal imbalance is particularly severe, and for both sexes their hormonal disruption can lead to high blood pressure and high cholesterol. Chronic pain is also a major concern, with most people over 50 suffering some joint problems, muscular problems, etc.

What amount should I aim for?

Over the age of 50 men and women alike should aim for 5mg per day. Again, although it is water soluble and you therefore must eat some every day, you only need to average 35mg per week to get enough.

When do I know I'm having enough?

Again, as many foods are fortified with B5 and as B5 is commonly found in animal and plant foods, it is incredibly rare for someone in a developed nation to have a B5 deficiency. However, if we are not eating enough calories, or enough variety of foods, it is possible to develop one. Both minor and serious B5 deficiencies display the same symptoms, which get more serious as the deficiency progresses. Fatigue, manic depressive symptoms, irritability, and insomnia are common mental health complaints in people with a vitamin B5 deficiency. They also experience stomach pains and vomiting, as well as burning sensations in their extremities and muscle cramping.

A particularly worrying symptom of vitamin B5 deficiency is upper respiratory infections. People over the age of 50 are more at risk of all respiratory infections, and are at serious risk of infections spreading and taking hold. This means that an upper respiratory infection can get into your lungs, and become severe enough as to hospitalize you. So, if you suspect vitamin B5 deficiency, don't hesitate to seek medical help.

You can definitely overdose on vitamin B5, and taking too much can cause diarrhea, bleeding, and other issues such as bad interactions with prescription drugs.

What foods can I find it in?

The very best food for B5 is once again liver, where a portion will give you three times the amount you need. Red meats and game in general provide an excellent amount of B5 too. However, there are still many plant based solutions, from avocado to sunflower seeds, where even small amounts of these foods can give you what you need. 2-3 ounces of seeds, for example, will give you your complete RDA.

When should I consider supplements?

Although deficiencies are rare, if you are on a hormonal supplement, have abused alcohol in the past or are currently doing so, have an intestinal disorder, or are on antibiotics, you may find yourself at increased risk of deficiency. Talk to your doctor about a supplement routine to suit your needs.

What do I need to be careful about?

Do not consume B5 supplements if you are on any other medication without help and support from your doctor, as they interact with many drugs.

Vitamin B6, Pyridoxine

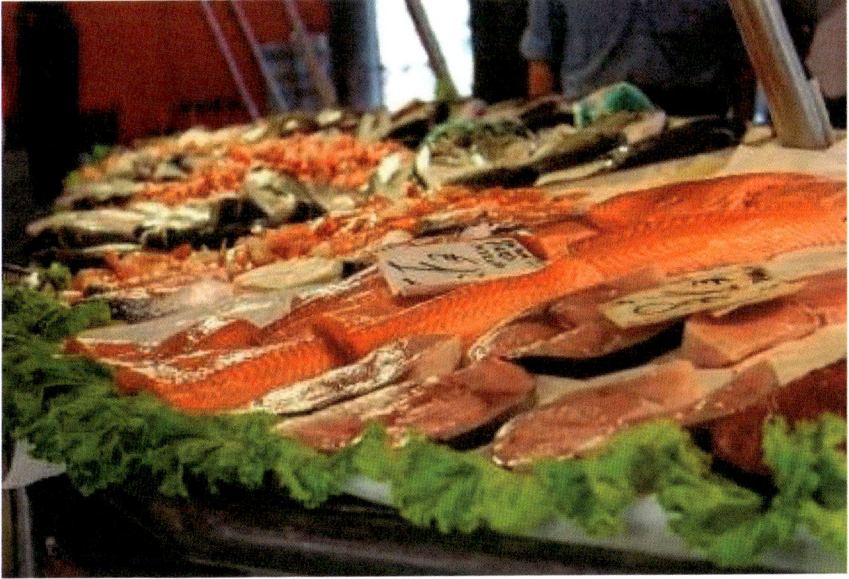

Soluble type: water.

What does it do?

There are many different types of B6, and all of them are very useful, working on improving our movement ability, memory and cognitive function, ATP creation from glucose and ketones, and healthy blood flow. It also is important in the development of hemoglobin in our red blood cells, maintaining an even mood, controlling pain, and controlling blood sugar. It even plays a role in strengthening our immune system!

How does it help people over the age of 50?

Vitamin B6 is crucial to every single bodily function, and having a wide range of different B6 vitamins is important as well. As our bodies tend to degrade as we grow older, the boosting effects of vitamin B6 are essential. Even more so when we consider that older people are prone to deficiencies.

What amount should I aim for?

Under the age of 50 most people are advised to take only 1.3 milligrams per day. But as we grow older we become much more vulnerable to B6 deficiencies. This is in part why older people get ill more often. So as adults over the age of 50, we must aim for 1.7 milligrams per day.

When do I know I'm having enough?

Vitamin B6 deficiency is incredibly unlikely in your youth, however it is very common in people aged 50 or over. Serious vitamin B6 deficiency in people over the age of 50 includes increased risk of heart disease, rheumatoid arthritis, and Alzheimer's disease. If you already have these conditions they will certainly get worse.

A mild vitamin B6 deficiency includes mood swings, confusion, aches and pains in our muscles, and suddenly developing poor energy, motivation, and strength. Many older people experience these symptoms anyway, as a consequence of illness or medications they are taking, so always keep an eye out for symptoms worsening suddenly, or developing out of the blue.

Vitamin B6 is impossible to overdose on naturally, but if you take supplements, or eat a large amount of foods like grains or energy drinks, which are often fortified with B6, you can get too much. A vitamin B6 overdose is not as severe as some other overdoses, but temporarily you will feel muscle numbness and confusion.

What foods can I find it in?

Like most B vitamins, B6 can be found in all muscle meats and fish. For a plant based option, most nuts and beans have plenty in them, as well as some seeds. Two interesting additions are avocado and blackstrap molasses, both very rich in vitamin B6.

When should I consider supplements?

As a person over the age of 50, it is worth talking to your doctor about supplements even if your diet is generally good and you have no health complaints.

What do I need to be careful about?

As it affects so much of your body, vitamin B6 can interact with a whole host of medications. Never start a B6 supplement regime without talking to your doctor first.

Vitamin B9, Folic Acid, Folate

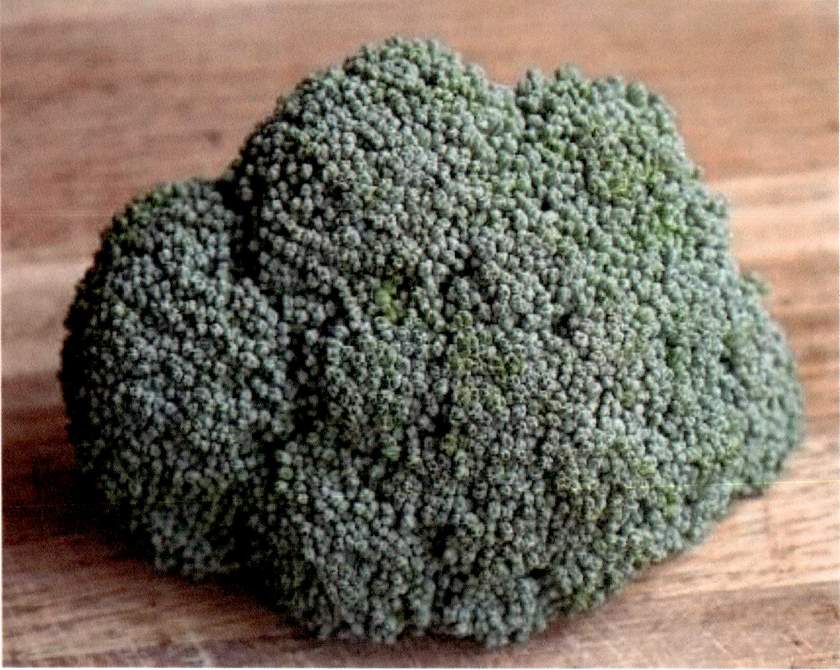

Soluble type: water.

What does it do?

Vitamin B9 plays a crucial role in copying and synthesizing DNA, which is why it is so essential to pregnant women, for example. It also has many different functions related to those of other B vitamins, such as ATP creation or immune system boosting.

How does it help people over the age of 50?

As we grow older the telomeres at the end of our chromosomes shorten. This damages our DNA, resulting in more and more errors happening as our cells split, and these mutations can lead to health complaints. Consuming enough vitamin B9 ensures that we can regenerate our cells as flawlessly as possible, keeping every organ in our bodies in better health for longer. This means vitamin B9 plays a role in preventing cancer, heart disease, and cognitive decline.

What amount should I aim for?

Adults need 400 micrograms of vitamin B9 per day to function optimally, however if your immune system is weak or you are suffering a condition that impacts your DNA and cell multiplication, for example cancer, you may benefit from more.

When do I know I'm having enough?

Vitamin B9 deficiency is very rare in developed nations, but it still happens. You are more at risk if you at some point in your life have abused alcohol, if you have a liver or kidney condition, or if you are on medication for diabetes or constipation. Symptoms of a serious deficiency include serious anemia, chronic fatigue or lethargy, and frequent, serious illness.

Symptoms of a minor deficiency are easier to miss. You will be ill a bit more often than usual, and more prone to irritability.

Your skin will be pale and lifeless in its complexion, and your hair may lose volume and color. And you will experience digestive issues such as constipation, bloating, and gut irritation. Ulcers and a sore tongue can also be a sign.

What foods can I find it in?

Vitamin B9 is found in leafy greens, organ meats, and beans. Therefore, if you are suffering a deficiency, you can often correct it with spinach, kale, broccoli, liver, or black beans. For a natural boost, wheat germ is particularly high in vitamin B9.

When should I consider supplements?

If you suffer liver or kidney dysfunctions, are being medicated for diabetes, or frequently take laxatives you may need a vitamin B9 supplement to keep your levels high enough.

What do I need to be careful about?

Research has found that even when we account for illness, physical condition, and medications, people absorb vitamin B9 very differently. Therefore, if you display symptoms of deficiency, do not hesitate to increase the amount of vitamin B9 foods you eat, or to ask your doctor about supplementation.

Vitamin B12, Cobalamin

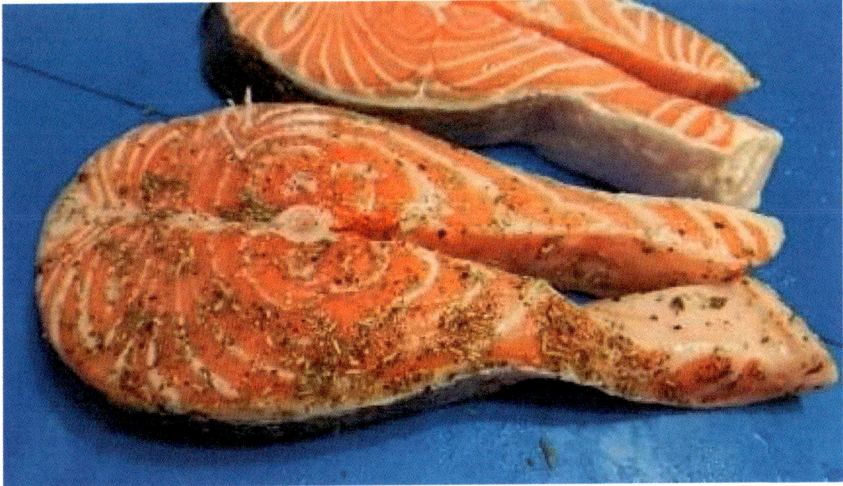

Soluble type: water.

What does it do?

Vitamin B12 is essential for producing digestive enzymes and ensuring that our cells receive the nutrients they need. It is required for over 100 different everyday bodily processes, such as synthesizing DNA, forming red blood cells, and boosting the immune system.

How does it help people over the age of 50?

As it affects every part of our bodies, adequate vitamin B12 intake is essential to live a longer, healthier, happier life.

41

What amount should I aim for?

Absorption varies from person to person, so aim for 1-2 servings of vitamin B12 rich foods every day.

When do I know I'm having enough?

This vitamin is a rare one where most people in developed nations *aren't* getting enough. Most of us do not eat diets which are complete or healthy enough for adequate vitamin B12 intake. But there are other reasons why you may be deficient. As we grow older we produce a lot less intrinsic factor in our stomachs. Intrinsic factor helps us absorb vitamin B12, so this drop could result in less vitamin B12 being absorbed. This is made worse if you take antacids regularly.

Deficiency usually shows the same signs, and each symptom varies from mild to severe depending on how deficient you are. Fatigue, lethargy, weakness, aches and pains, memory loss, cognitive decline, and mood changes are all common. This deficiency will also wear down your cardiovascular system, causing shortness of breath, and your gut, causing cramping, nausea, and diarrhea.

It is impossible to have too much vitamin B12. Firstly, because it is a water-soluble vitamin and therefore it does not build up in our body. And secondly because it metabolizes so slowly that even if we were to consume an overdose of it, if we are healthy our bodies will eliminate the excess long before we reached critical levels.

What foods can I find it in?

Animal produce are our main sources of it. Organ meats are the highest, followed by fish, then dairy, then lean and white meats.

When should I consider supplements?

Vitamin B12 shots are the most viable sort of supplement available. If you have any condition which means you may not absorb B12 well, such as pernicious anemia, then you could need an annual vitamin B12 shot. If you are vegan you could also do with one, as most people do not properly metabolize plant based vitamin B12 sources.

What do I need to be careful about?

As a final note about the B vitamins, it is a very good idea to consume them all together. In natural sources, they can all be found together, and they interact with each other in the blood stream. As they are not stored very well, consuming them all in one go promotes these interactions and ensures they all do their best job.

Vitamin C

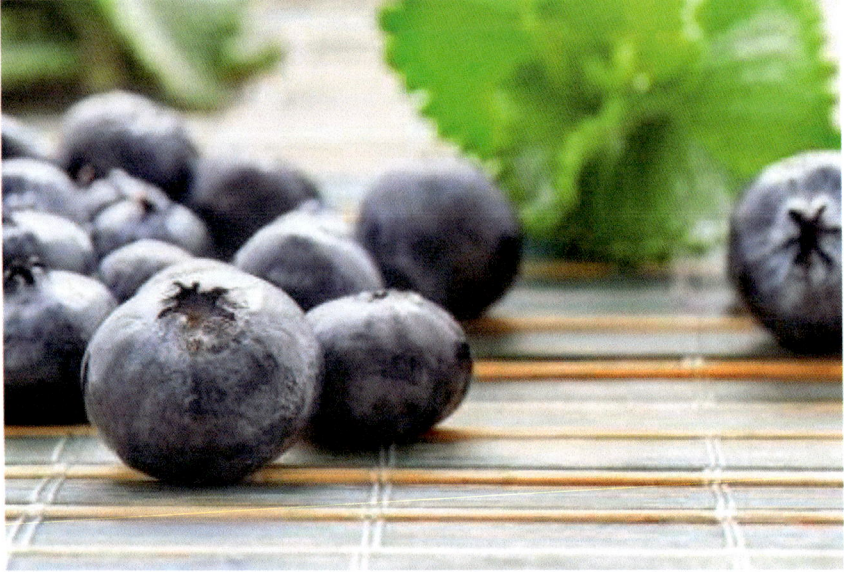

Soluble type: water.

What does it do?

Vitamin C plays many essential roles in our body. Even though it gets credit for fighting colds, in reality its major role is preventing them by supporting our immune system. It is also essential for fortifying our bones, and as an antioxidant is crucial to slowing down cell damage. It is needed for absorbing iron too.

How does it help people over the age of 50?

As we grow older our immune systems weaken and cell regrowth slows down. Vitamin C can help protect us against a weaker immune system and improve the rate at which our cells replenish themselves. It also reverses the oxidation done by free radicals, reversing the ageing process.

What amount should I aim for?

Men and women alike benefit from 50mg per day, although a little more can always help.

When do I know I'm having enough?

As vitamin C is a water-soluble vitamin, its levels decline slowly but surely as soon as we stop eating it. Early on in your deficiency the symptoms are subtler. You will notice that your blood flow is excessive, above all. You bruise easily, your gums swell and bleed, your nose bleeds, etc. You will also notice you get more colds than usual.

If you allow your vitamin C levels to remain low, you put yourself at risk of scurvy. Scurvy results in serious skin and clotting complaints, as well as high blood pressure, damage to your gallbladder, atherosclerosis, and a whole host of cancers. Vitamin C overdose, especially from whole foods, is unheard of and should not concern you.

What foods can I find it in?

Fruits, especially citrus fruits and berries, are very rich in vitamin C. But vitamin C breaks down when cooked or left too long, so make sure to eat your fruits and vegetables fresh and raw for the most vitamin C intake.

When should I consider supplements?

As we grow older our guts become much more sensitive, making some foods impossible to eat. If you find you cannot eat much fruit due to digestive upsets, then you may need a supplement.

What do I need to be careful about?

Just as vitamin C improves iron absorption, it has been hypothesized that the relationship works the other way around too. So always take vitamin C and iron supplements together, just in case.

Vitamin D2 and D3

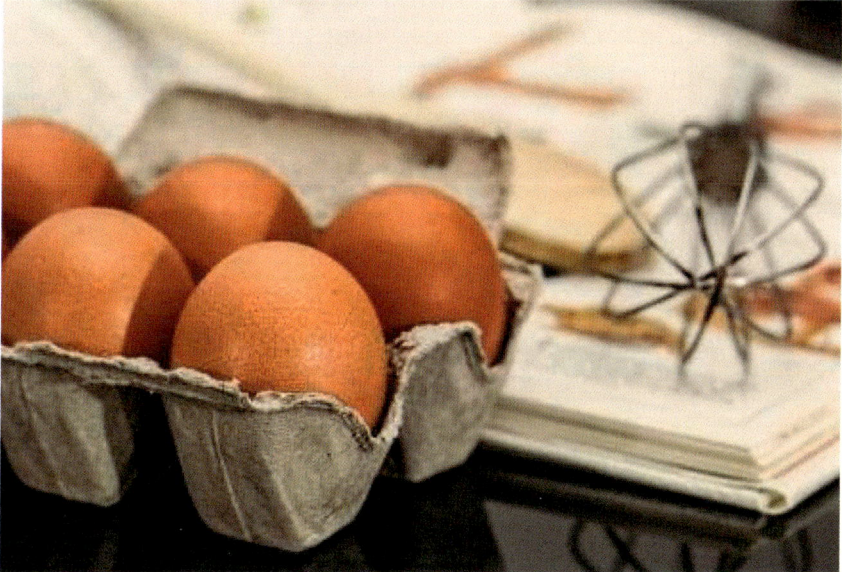

Soluble type: fat.

What does it do?

Vitamin D plays three key roles in our bodies. The first and simplest is bone development. Vitamin D is essential to absorbing and using calcium properly. But vitamin D is also vital for maintaining a healthy hormonal balance and regulating our moods. Those last two functions naturally have an effect on our general health and wellbeing.

How does it help people over the age of 50?

As we grow older we are at risk of a whole host of conditions. Osteoporosis, depression, and hormonal imbalances are common complaints. For women over the age of 50, these are particularly marked. By ensuring we have enough vitamin D we can avoid the worst of these conditions.

What amount should I aim for?

Because it is more a hormone than a vitamin, vitamin D is measured in international units, or IU. We need 400 IU of vitamin D a day, minimum, to do well.

When do I know I'm having enough?

As long as you get daily exposure to sunlight, you are guaranteed to get enough vitamin D. Just getting 20 minutes of sun on your skin can help you make 20,000 IU, and as it is fat soluble you can store a lot of that, giving you plenty. However, in the Northern Hemispheres you are at risk of deficiency, due to long and cold winters.

Signs of deficiency include frequent illness, low mood, lethargy and fatigue, and general weakness. These symptoms get progressively worse as the deficiency develops, culminating in clinical depression and even neurological disorders. Long term deficiency also causes rickets and osteoporosis. There is no known way to overdose on vitamin D.

What foods can I find it in?

Vitamin D3 is the only vitamin our bodies can spontaneously make, all on their own, with just a little sunlight. In that respect, it is more like a hormone than a vitamin. Twenty minutes with a third of your skin exposed to sunlight provides 20,000 IU of D3. However, vitamin D2, a vitamin D3 precursor, is edible, and can be found in eggs and seafood.

When should I consider supplements?

If you cannot get sun on your skin for at least five minutes a day, three days a week, you may need a supplement. Also, if you are a dark-skinned person living in a cold climate you may need a supplement too, as melanin inhibits vitamin D3 production.

What do I need to be careful about?

Vitamin D2 in supplements, and fortified milks including cow's milk and various vegan milks, is not as useable as vitamin D3 from sunlight, so you will need a higher dose.

Vitamin E

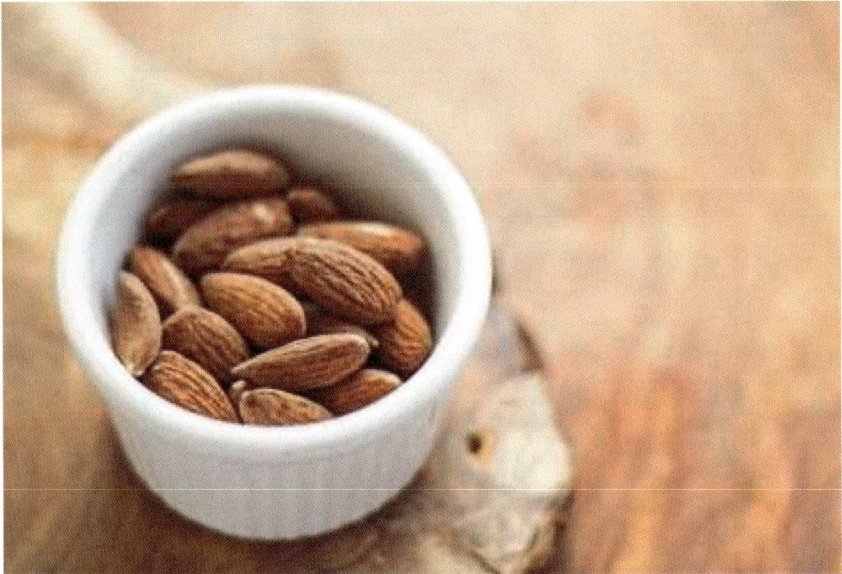

Soluble type: fat.

What does it do?

Vitamin E is nature's most powerful antioxidant, reversing the effects of ageing by stopping free radicals from damaging our cells. This means that vitamin E can prevent and treat cardiovascular disease, improve skin health and appearance, and keep our organs strong and healthy. This means a reduced risk of high blood pressure, hardened arteries, heart attacks, cancer, liver disease, and kidney failure.

How does it help people over the age of 50?

Our whole lives, free radicals are continually attacking the cells in our bodies. This damage builds up over the years, and gets progressively worse. By consuming enough vitamin E, we can slow, halt, or even reverse some of this damage, reversing the effects of ageing and increasing our longevity. It has also been found to slow the development of Alzheimer's.

What amount should I aim for?

Adults need around 15 milligrams of vitamin E per day, although as it is fat soluble it is perfectly possible to eat a lot of it and go a short while with a reduced intake.

When do I know I'm having enough?

Until recently it was assumed that as most diets are rich in vitamin E and as vitamin E requirements are so low, deficiencies must be rare, and caused largely by illness, not by diet. However, it has come to light that people absorb vitamin E at different rates, and that many diets truly are deficient in vitamin E of all kinds.

Vitamin E deficiency is made even worse by poor fat absorption. Vitamin E is a fat-soluble vitamin, so if we do not eat enough fat, or do not absorb fat well, we will become deficient in it. So, if you have trouble with your pancreas, gallbladder, or have had gastric bypass surgery, you may become deficient.

Symptoms of vitamin E deficiency include loss of muscle coordination, eyesight troubles, and trouble speaking.

Vitamin E poisoning is very much possible, and for this reason it is not recommended to eat over 1000mg per day. If you have a serious deficiency your doctor may prescribe you a very high dose up to this amount, but more than this causes complications in most people. The most severe consequences are heart attacks in people with diabetes, strokes, development and worsening of bleeding disorders, and making it so that cancers in regression may return.

What foods can I find it in?

The best possible foods for vitamin E are nuts and seeds. A cupful of sunflower seeds, almonds, hazelnuts, or wheat germ will provide more than enough vitamin E for one day. And many fruits, like mangoes, avocados, kiwis, and tomatoes are also high in vitamin E, although not as much as nuts and seeds are.

When should I consider supplements?

Synthetic edible vitamin E has been found to not provide the same benefits as natural vitamin E, so it is not advisable to take supplements. Instead, focus on eating a rich and varied diet high in both raw and cooked plants. However, if you cannot absorb enough fat to keep your vitamin E levels up, it is worth considering supplements that are applied to the skin, as it is possible to absorb vitamin E through our skin in large enough amounts to avoid deficiency.

What do I need to be careful about?

There are actually eight different types of vitamin E, all of which coming from different food sources and providing their own unique benefits. They can be divided into two groups, tocotrienols and tocopherols. It has been found that too much tocopherol vitamin E can stop you absorbing tocotrienols as well, which can lead to deficiency symptoms even in people who are consuming enough. For this reason, eat a wide variety of fruit, vegetables, nuts and seeds. Rice oil, rice bran oil, and palm oil are particularly high in tocotrienol vitamin Es.

Vitamin K, Biotin, B7

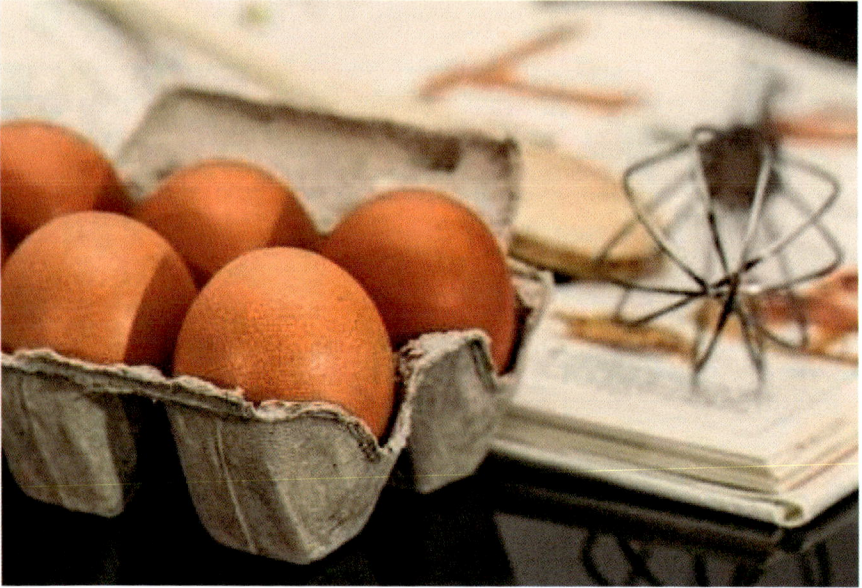

Soluble type: water.

What does it do?

Biotin, officially vitamin B7, is often nicknamed vitamin H due to its benefits to Haar und Haut (Hair and Hide, or Hair and Skin). It is a coenzyme that helps us to metabolize glucose and ketones into ATP, and strengthens keratins and collagen in our skin, hair, and nails, resulting in improved health and appearance of these body parts.

How does it help people over the age of 50?

We tend to think of our skin as a cosmetic issue, but it serves a number of vital functions, such as retaining moisture, defending our bodies against bacteria, and protecting us from UV damage. As we age our skin weakens, so consuming enough vitamin H can help us to strengthen our skin and keep us healthy.

What amount should I aim for?

You need to eat 30 micrograms of vitamin H every day. As it is absorbed and processed poorly, you need to try and consume this daily without fail to ensure you get enough.

When do I know I'm having enough?

Vitamin H deficiencies are very rare, but they do happen. Initial symptoms are a sudden loss of energy, muscle and gut cramps, tingling in our arms and legs, and mood swings. As the deficiency progresses we find that our skin and hair dry our and our skin becomes sensitive. Our hair will become brittle and fall out and our muscles will become very sore. In the end, we can see nerve damage and cognitive impairment caused by our brain tissue becoming damaged due to lack of energy.

People at risk of a vitamin H deficiency usually have some form of gut imbalance. People on antibiotics and some anti-seizure medications find their gut balance is disrupted and their absorption of vitamin H is limited.

People with gut conditions like celiac, leaky gut, or IBS are also at risk of deficiency. However, if you suffer any sort of intestinal disruption on a regular basis you are at risk of deficiency.

As vitamin H is water soluble and very poorly absorbed and stored, there is no risk of overdosing on it. No matter how much of it we eat, we will only metabolize as much as we need, and any small excesses will be passed out in our urine long before our blood levels could become dangerous.

What foods can I find it in?

Biotin is contained in almost every food, from meat to cheese, from eggs to berries, from cauliflower to grains. However, some have more than others, with liver and eggs being particularly rich sources. That said, we need so little that even a slice of whole grain bread will give you all you need.

When should I consider supplements?

When you have any gut disruption at all, whether it is an illness, due to diet, or yet to be diagnosed, talk to your doctor about a vitamin H, or vitamin B7, supplement to ensure that your health is not affected.

What do I need to be careful about?

When choosing a supplement, bear in mind there are many different sources of vitamin H, and that only the natural sources have proven benefits, with all artificial versions being of questionable quality.

Vitamin K

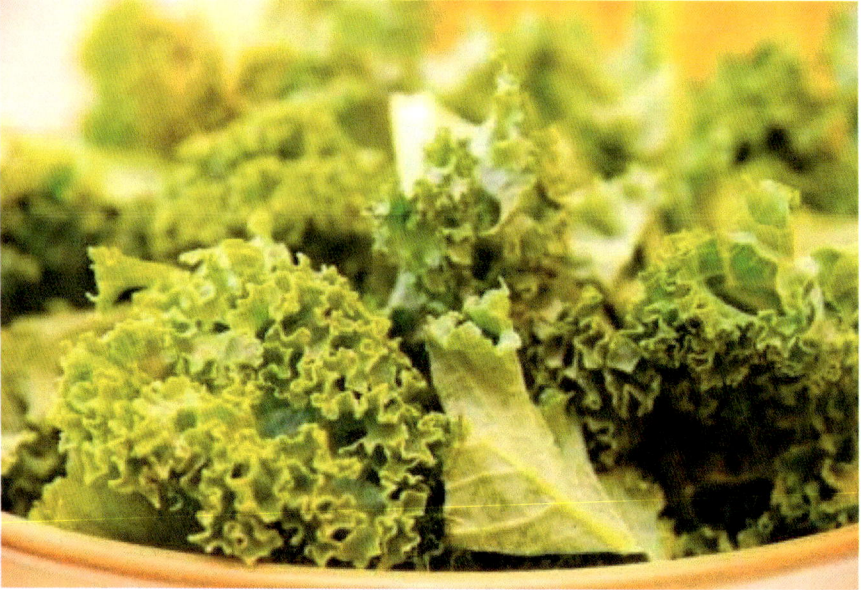

Soluble type: fat.

What does it do?

Vitamin K's two most important roles are in growing and replenishing our bones, and in promoting heart health and blood clotting.

How does it help people over the age of 50?

For people over the age of fifty, heart and bone health are very important. Ensuring your heart and bones retain much of the strength they had in your youth will keep you active, pain free, and happy, for much longer.

What amount should I aim for?

You are recommended to eat 90 micrograms per day, however as it is fat soluble you can go a while without eating any, thanks to your own reserves, and then stock up again later.

When do I know I'm having enough?

A vitamin K deficiency becomes obvious at first when we notice abnormal bleeding. Suddenly bruising very badly for no reason at all, nose bleeds, or bleeding from the gums with no sign of mouth infection, can be signs you are deficient.

Whilst a vitamin K overdose is not possible for healthy people, if you have any sort of clotting disorder or heart condition you will find that too much vitamin K will make you very ill.

What foods can I find it in?

As it is produced by the bacteria in your gut, any food which feeds your guts, such as leafy greens or dairy, will guarantee you an amount. A single cup of Swiss chard provides all the vitamin K you need.

When should I consider supplements?

If you have a gut condition, osteoporosis, or a clotting condition, then talk to your doctor about supplementing.

Also, beware having vitamin K and vitamin E supplements at once, as they can cancel each other out.

What do I need to be careful about?

How much vitamin K you have depends entirely on your gut health. If you suffer from any gut-based condition, then you need to check your vitamin K levels, as you may be deficient. This means that someone with celiac may suffer bleeding in the gut, which decreases their vitamin K, which makes the bleeding worse. So, talk to your doctor about breaking the cycle.

Final Thoughts

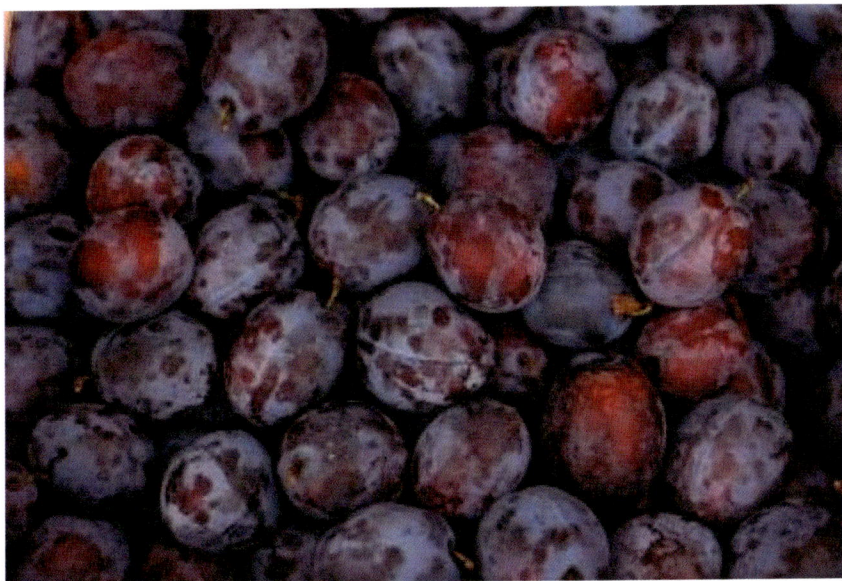

Sometimes we also need to consider whether vitamins are not being processed properly. In rare cases, the cause of a vitamin deficiency is not that we aren't consuming enough of the vitamin, but that we are not absorbing enough of it, or able to use the amount that is in our blood. We have already explored how some nutrients work together to ensure that the other one works properly.

But we also need to bear in mind that we rely on enzymes and bacteria to extract these nutrients, and red blood cells to carry them where they are needed. If you are eating the right foods in the right amounts, or even taking vitamin supplements, and still experiencing low vitamin symptoms, it is time to talk with your doctor.

It is common in these cases that an organ is not working properly, and this is causing your vitamin levels to stay low no matter how many vitamins you eat. It's a bit like making a plate of food versus eating it. Your plate can have all the right things on it, but if they don't go into you they're useless.

Likewise, you can put all the right things into your body, but if your body can't extract the vitamins, they're useless. Often vitamin malabsorption is a sign of an illness starting, or an organ failing, so don't hesitate to contact your doctor as it could even save your life.

About the Author

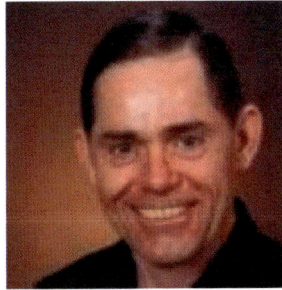

I have published over 125 books on Amazon for Kindle, CreateSpace and other publishing platforms.

While most of my books are on health and fitness in general, as I age (now 65) at the time of this writing) my topics of interest are geared toward aging baby boomers and older.

Besides my own writing, I also ghostwrite ebooks, books, reports, articles, blogs and do Kindle conversions for clients on a variety of topics.

Today my wife and I are retired from our careers and live in Gold Canyon, AZ. I now write as a retirement business where you'll find me happily sitting in my office typing away on my laptop as I work on my next book or ghostwriting project . . . that is if we are not traveling on a cruise ship - our new-found mode of travel.

Printed in Great Britain
by Amazon